The Basic Essentials

D0456193

FIRST AID
FOR THE OUTDOORS

By William W. Forgey, M.D.

ICS BOOKS, Inc.
Merrillville, Indiana

THE BASIC ESSENTIALS OF
FIRST AID FOR THE OUTDOORS

1st Printing11-89, 2nd Printing 5-94
3rd Printing11-94, 4th Printing 3-95
5th Printing 4-96

10 9 8 7 6

Printed in U.S.A.

DEDICATION

To Tom Whittaker and all of the members of the Cooperative Wilderness Handicapped Outdoor Group, the famous CW Hogs of Idaho State University, who have demonstrated their true love and appreciation of the outdoors, this book is fondly dedicated.*

*For further information on the outdoor education program at Idaho State University, and for information about the significant pro-gramming afforded handicapped individuals through the CW HOG program, contact Tom Whittaker, Idaho State University, Campus Recreation, Box 8105, Pocatello, ID 83209, (208) 236-0211.

Published by:
ICS BOOKS, Inc.
1370 E. 86th. Place
Merrillville, IN. 46410

recycled paper

All ICS titles are printed on 50% recycled paper from pre-consumer waste. All sheets are processed without using acid.

Library of Congress Cataloging-in-Publication Data

Forgey, William W., 1942-
    First aid for the outdoors : the basic essentials / by William W.
Forgey.
        p.   cm. -- (The Basic essentials series)
    Bibliography: p.
    Includes index.
    ISBN 0-934802-43-2 : $4.95
    1. Outdoor life--Accidents and injuries. 2. First aid in illness
and injury. 3. Medical emergencies. I. Title.
RC88.9.095F67   1989
616.02'52--dc19
                                                                88-32997
                                                                CIP

TABLE OF CONTENTS

1. WILDERNESS WOUND CARE

The most common outdoor injury that you will have to treat will be friction blisters and minor thermal burns. These injuries always occur early in the trip. New equipment will rub, and let's face it — when cooking over a campfire, many of us forget just how hot that pot has become. At least we learn quickly and veteran campers will soon only remember burned fingers and blistered feet, rather than continue to experience them.

Friction Blisters

A relatively new and easily obtainable substance has revolutionized the prevention and care of friction blisters. The substance is Spenco 2nd Skin, available at most athletic supply and drug stores. Made from an inert, breathable gel consisting of 4% polyethylene oxide and 96% water, it has the feel and consistency of, well most people would say snot. It comes in various sized sheets, sterile and sealed in water-tight packages. It is very cool to the touch, in fact large sheets are sold to cover infants to reduce a fever. It has three valuable properties that make it so useful. One, it will remove all friction between two moving surfaces (hence its use in prevention) and two, it cleans and deodorizes wounds by absorbing blood, serum, or pus. Three, its cooling effect is very soothing, which aids in pain relief.

After opening the sealed package, you will find the Spenco 2nd Skin sandwiched between two sheets of cellophane. Remove the cellophane from the side which will be applied to the wound or hot spot. It must be secured to the wound and for that purpose the same company produces an adhesive knit bandage.

For treatment of a hot spot, remove the cellophane from one side and apply this gooey side against the wound, again securing it with the knit bandaging. If a friction blister has developed, it will have to be lanced. Cleanse with soap or surgical scrub and open along an edge with a #11 scalpel blade or equal. See figure 1. After expressing the fluid, apply a fully stripped piece of 2nd Skin. This is done by removing the cellophane from one side, then applying it to the wound. Once on the skin surface, remove the cellophane from the outside edge. Over this you will need to place the adhesive knit. The bandage must be kept moist with clean water. Applied through the adhesive knit, routine moistening will allow the same bandage to be used for days or until the wound is healed.

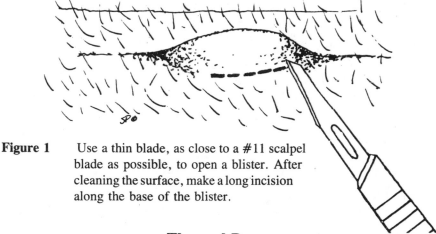

Figure 1   Use a thin blade, as close to a #11 scalpel blade as possible, to open a blister. After cleaning the surface, make a long incision along the base of the blister.

Thermal Burns

As soon as possible remove the source of the burn — quick immersion into cool water will help eliminate additional heat from scalding water or burning fuels and clothing. Or otherwise suffocate the flames with clothing, sand, etc.

Treatment of burns depends upon the extent (percent of the body covered) and the depth (degree) of the injury. The percent of the body covered is estimated by referring to the Rule of Nines, as indicated in figure 2. For example: an entire arm equals 9% of the body surface area, therefore the burn of just one side of the forearm would equal about 2%. The proportions are slightly different for children.

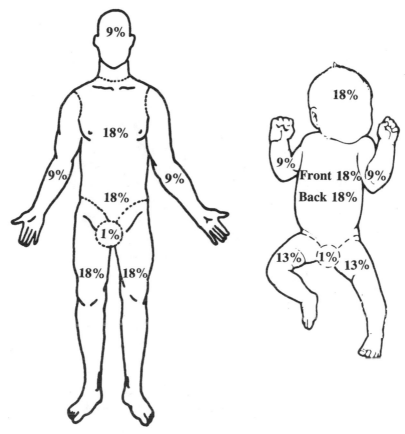

Figure 2   The Rule of Nines helps determine the percentage of a body covered by burns. Note the slight difference between an adult and child.

Severity of burns is indicated by degree. First Degree (superficial) will have redness and be dry and painful. Second Degree (partial skin thickness) will be moist, painful, and have blister formation with reddened bases. Third Degree (deep) involves the full thickness of the skin and extends into the underlying tissue with char, loss of substance, or discoloration. These are frequently not painful due to nerve destruction, although there will be painful lesions of second and first degree burn surrounding the area. See figure 3.

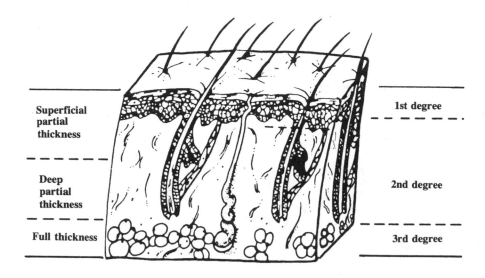

Figure 3   Burn thickness and degree. 1st degree: only epidermis involvement; 2nd degree: blisters separate the epidermis from lower dermal layers; 3rd degree: destruction of dermis and below.

The field treatment of burns has also been revolutionized by the development of Spenco 2nd Skin. It is the perfect substance to use on 1st, 2nd, or 3rd degree burns. Its cooling effect relieves pain, while its sterile covering absorbs fluid easily from the wound. If applied to a charred 3rd degree burn, it provides a sterile cover that does not have to be changed. When the patient arrives at a hospital, it can easily be removed in a whirlpool bath.

Burn patients can generally be managed quite well by the first aider if they are not worse than 2nd degree and as long as they do not cover more than 15% of the body surface area of an adult (10% of a child). Burns more extensive than this, and burns which involve the face or include more than one joint of the hand, are best treated professionally. The first aid treatment will be as above, but additionally, treat for shock and arrange evacuation.

Shock Care

Injury care, whether in the wilderness or not, can be broken into chronological phases. The first phase consists of SAVING THE VICTIM'S LIFE — by stopping the bleeding and treating for shock. Even if the victim is not bleeding, you will want to treat for shock. Shock has many fancy medical definitions, but on the bottom line it amounts to an inadequate oxygenated blood supply

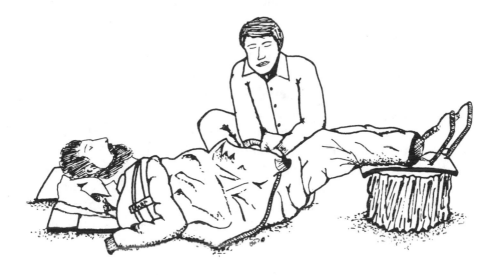

Figure 4   The shock treatment position includes lowering the head and raising the extremities. Always protect the patient from the environment with a covering and under-padding.

getting to the head. Complete discussions of shock can be found in references 1, 5, and 10. Lay the patient down, elevate feet above the head, and provide protection from the environment — from both the ground and the atmosphere. Grab anything which you can find for this at first — use jackets, pack frames, unrolled tents, whatever. See figure 4. Patients with head injuries are best allowed to have slight head elevation, unless concern for a neck injury exists. Immobilization of the patient with an injured neck to prevent spinal cord damage is essential.

Lacerations

Direct pressure is the best method of stopping bleeding — in fact pressure alone can stop bleeding from amputated limbs! When the accident first occurs, you may even need to use your bare hand to stem the flow of blood. This direct pressure may have to be applied 5, 10, even 30 minutes. Apply it as long as it takes! With the blood stopped, even if only with your hand, and the victim on the ground in the shock treatment position, the actual emergency is over. Their life is safe. And you have bought time to gather together various items you need to perform the definitive job of caring for this wound. You have also treated for psychogenic shock — the shock of "fear." For obviously someone knows what to do: they have taken charge, they have stopped the bleeding, they are giving orders to gather materials together. The shock caused by fear is more of a problem than that caused by loss of blood.

In the first aid management of this wound, the next step is simply bandaging and then transporting the victim to professional medical care. Further care of a wound takes the practitioner beyond the first aid phase. It is generally best to seek professional help for aggressive wound cleansing and closure technique. Trip leaders requiring this knowledge may find detailed information in reference 5.

Abrasions

An abrasion is the loss of surface skin due to a scraping injury. The best treatment is cleansing with Hibiclens surgical scrub, application of triple antibiotic ointment, and the use of Spenco 2nd Skin with Adhesive Knit Bandage — all components of the the Outdoor First Aid Kit listed in Appendix B. This type of wound oozes profusely, but the above bandaging allows rapid healing, excellent protection, and considerable pain relief. Avoid the use of alcohol on these wounds as it tends to damage the tissue, to say nothing of causing excessive pain. Lacking first aid supplies, cleanse gently with mild detergent and protect from dirt, bugs, etc., the best that you can. Tetanus immunization should have been within 10 years.

Puncture Wounds

Allow puncture wounds to bleed, thus hoping to effect an automatic irrigation of bacteria from the wound. If available, apply

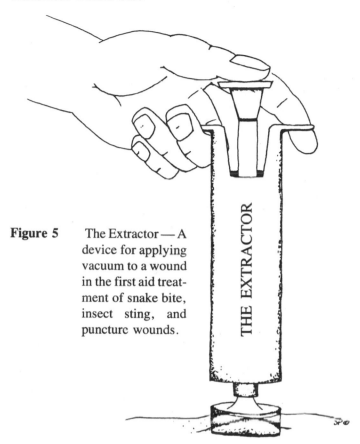

Figure 5 The Extractor — A device for applying vacuum to a wound in the first aid treatment of snake bite, insect sting, and puncture wounds.

THE EXTRACTOR

suction with the Extractor (venom suction device) immediately and continue the vacuum for 20 to 30 minutes. The Extractor, see figure 5, is recommended for inclusion in your Outdoor First Aid Kit (Appendix B). Cleanse the wound area with surgical scrub — or soapy water — and apply triple antibiotic ointment to the surrounding skin surface. Do not tape shut, but rather start warm compress applications for 20 minutes, every 2 hours for the next 2 days. These soaks should be as warm as the patient can tolerate without danger of burning the skin. Larger pieces of cloth work best — such as undershirts — as they hold the heat longer. Dressings should be with a clean cloth. If sterile items are in short supply, they need not be used on this type of wound. Use clean cloths, or boil such items and allow to cool and dry before use. Tetanus immunization should have been within 5 years for dirty injuries such as puncture wounds. The person may safely wait until they get home if their last tetanus immunization was within the past 10 years.

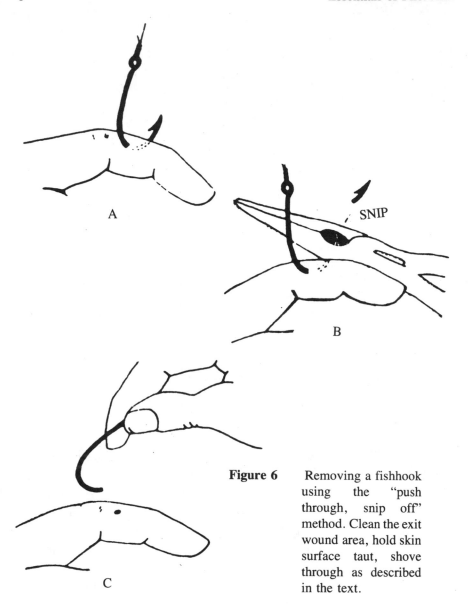

Figure 6   Removing a fishhook using the "push through, snip off" method. Clean the exit wound area, hold skin surface taut, shove through as described in the text.

Fishhook Removal

There are three basic methods of removing a fishhook.

Push through, snip off method: As outlined in figure 6, the steps are simple: A) Push the hook through, B) snip it off, C) back the barb-less hook out, D) treat the puncture wounds. While the technique seems straightforward, consider a few points: 1) Pushing the hook should not endanger underlying or adjacent structures.

This limits the technique's usefulness, but it is still frequently an easy, quick method to employ. 2) Skin is not easy to push through. It is very elastic and will tent up over the barb as you try to push it through. Place side-cutting wire cutters, with jaws spread apart, over the point on the surface where you expect the hook point to punch through. 3) This is a painful process and skin hurts when being poked from the bottom up, as much as from the top down. Once committed, get the push through portion of this project over with in a hurry. 4) This adds a second puncture wound to the victim's anatomy. Cleanse the skin at the anticipated penetration site before shoving the hook through using soap or a surgical scrub. 5) When snipping the protruding point off, cover the wound area with your free hand to protect you and others from the flying hook point. Otherwise you may need to refer to the section on "removing foreign bodies from the eye."

Figure 7   The "string jerk" method of fishhook removal. Push the shank handle to the skin surface, then pull a wrapped string along the surface to disengage the barb and remove the hook.

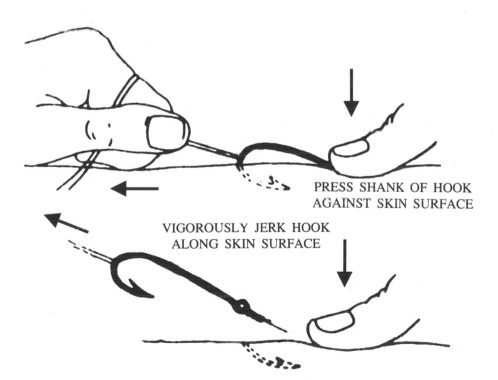

PRESS SHANK OF HOOK AGAINST SKIN SURFACE

VIGOROUSLY JERK HOOK ALONG SKIN SURFACE

The string jerk method: works best in areas with little connective tissue in the involved area. Fingers are loaded with fibrous tissue that tends to hinder a smooth hook removal. This technique works best in the back of the head, the shoulder, and most aspects of the torso, arms, and legs. It is highly useful and can be virtually painless, causing minimal trauma.

Important to the method is looping a line, such as the fish line, around the hook and insuring that this line is held flush against the skin. Pushing down on the eye portion of the hook helps disengage the hook barb, so that the quick pull will jerk the hook free with minimal trauma. See figure 7. Many times a victim has been quoted as asking *"When are you going to pull it out?"* after the job has been completed.

The dissection method: This technique, using either a hypodermic needle or a #11 scalpel blade, is illustrated in my book *Wilderness Medicine*, but should be reserved for instances of isolation with no hope of reaching professional help for several days.

Hooks which cannot be removed by the snip off or string jerk method should be taped in place, the fish line removed, and the patient evacuated to help. Avoid snipping the hook off near the skin surface, as this makes the physician's task of removal potentially more difficult. Place some triple antibiotic ointment on the wound site twice daily until help can be reached.

Splinter Removal

Prepare the wound with Hibiclens surgical scrub, soapy water, or other cleansing solution that does not discolor the skin. Minute splinters are hard enough to see without discoloring the skin and disguising them even more. If the splinter is shallow, or the point buried, use a needle or #11 scalpel blade (figure 1) to tease the tissue over the splinter to remove this top layer. The splinter can then be pried out.

It is best to be aggressive in removing this top layer and obtaining a substantial bite on the splinter with the splinter forceps (or tweezers), rather than nibbling off the end while making futile attempts to remove with inadequate exposure. When using the splinter forceps, grasp the instrument between the thumb and forefinger, resting the instrument on the middle finger and further resting the entire hand against the victim's skin, if necessary, to prevent tremor. Scc figure 8. Approach the splinter from the side, if exposed, grasping it as low as possible. Apply triple antibiotic afterwards.

Figure 8   Hold splinter forceps or tweezer parallel to the skin surface and grasp the splinter only after obtaining an adequate exposure by unroofing it adequately.

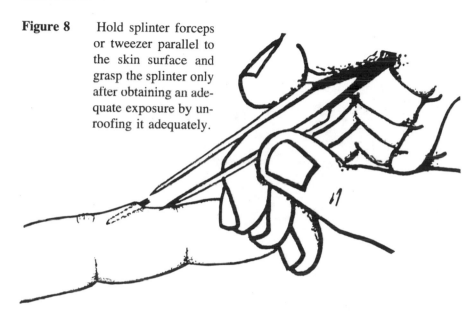

Tetanus immunization should be current within 10 years, or if a dirty wound, within 5 years. If the wound was dirty, scrub afterwards with Hibiclens or soapy water. If deep, treat as indicated above under PUNCTURE WOUND with hot soaks and antibiotic as indicated.

2. EYE, EAR, NOSE, MOUTH

No portion of our general well being affects us as much as our five senses, and four of them relate to proper function of the above organs.

Eye

The most common eye problems in the wilderness will be foreign body, abrasion, and infection (conjunctivitis). Therapy for these problems is virtually the same, except that it is very important to remove any foreign body that may be present.

Foreign Body

A calm, careful examination is necessary to adequately examine the eye for a foreign body. Very carefully shine a small light at the cornea (the surface of the eye above the pupil and iris) from one side to see if a minute speck becomes visible. By moving the light back and forth, one might see movement of a shadow on the iris of the eye and thus confirm the presence of a foreign body. A shadow that consistently stays put with blinking is probably a foreign body.

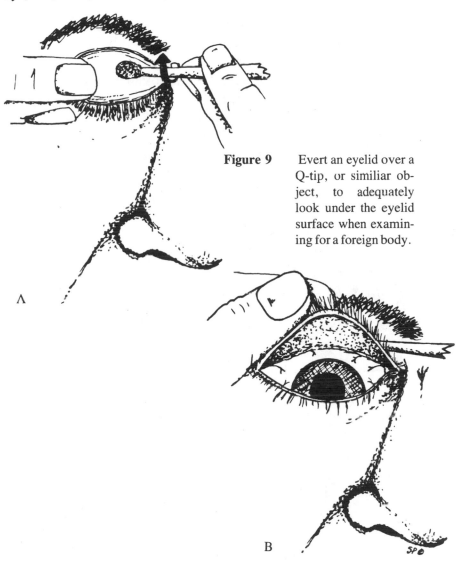

Figure 9 Evert an eyelid over a Q-tip, or similiar object, to adequately look under the eyelid surface when examining for a foreign body.

A

B

In making the foreign body examination, also be sure to check under the eyelids. Evert the upper lid over a Q-tip stick, thus examining not only the eyeball, but also the under-surface of the eyelid. See figure 9. This surface may be gently brushed with the cotton applicator to eliminate minute particles. Always use a fresh Q-tip when touching the eye or eyelid each additional time.

When a foreign body has been found, it can frequently be rinsed off with running water. Onc method is for the victim to hold their face under water and blink their eyes. Sometimes it can be easily prodded off with the edge of a clean cloth, such as a bandana.

Leave stubborn foreign bodies for removal by a physician in all but the most desperate circumstances. The patient should be evacuated to a physician at once, if at all possible. If you are stuck in the bush and have a difficult time removing an obvious foreign body from the surface of the cornea, a wait of two to three days may allow the cornea to ulcerate slightly so that removal by gentle prodding with a Q-tip handle may be *much* easier. Deeply lodged foreign bodies will have to be left for surgical removal.

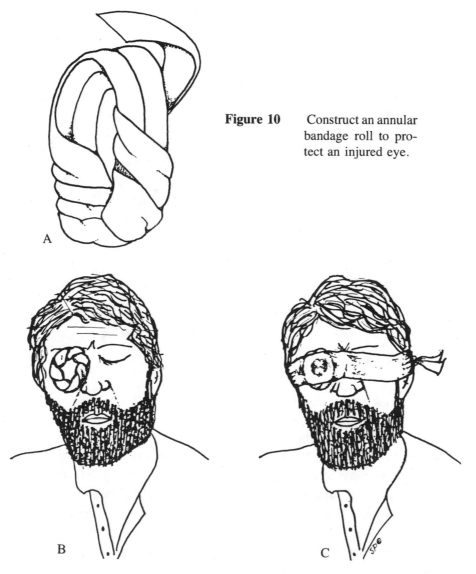

Figure 10   Construct an annular bandage roll to protect an injured eye.

Patching the eye will help alleviate pain. Patch techniques for the eye must allow for gentle closure of the eyelid and retard blinking activity. Generally both eyes must be patched for this to succeed. Simple strips of tape taping the eyelids shut may suffice. In case of trauma, a ring of cloth may be constructed to pad the eye without pressure over the eyeball. See figure 10. A simple eye patch with over-size gauze or cloth may work fine, as the bone of the orbital rim around the eye acts to protect the eyeball which is recessed. Try to avoid patching both eyes, except at times when the patient is resting. If eye drops are available they can provide some relief, but antibiotic drops are prescription medications. Seek professional help for any eye condition as soon as possible.

Eye Abrasion

Carefully examine the eye surface to insure that no foreign body is present. Check under the eyelids as indicated above. An abrasion on the eye will feel like a foreign body is present. Treat with soothing eye drops if available. Patch for comfort as indicated above.

Eye Infection

An infection of the eye will be heralded by a scratchy feeling, almost indistinguishable from a foreign body in the eye. The sclera or white of the eye will be reddened. Generally the eye will be matted shut in the morning with pus or granular matter.

Rinse with clean water frequently during the day. Eye infections such as common bacterial conjunctivitis, the most common infection, are self limiting and will generally clear themselves within two weeks. They can become much worse, however, so medical attention should be sought. Do not patch, but protect the eyes from sunlight. When one eye is infected, treat both eyes as the infection spreads easily to the non-infected eye.

Eye infections should be treated with a prescription antibiotic. As a temporary measure, various soothing eye drops and ointments are available without prescription, such as have been included in the recommended medical kit (Appendix B). If nasal congestion is also present, treatment with a decongestant, such as Actifed, is quite appropriate.

Ear

Pain in the ear can be associated with a number of sources. The history of trauma will be an obvious source of pain. Most ear pain is due to an *otitis media* or infection behind the ear drum (tympanic membrane), *otitis externa* or infection in the outer ear canal (auditory canal), or due to infection elsewhere (generally a dental infection, infected tonsil, or lymph node in the neck near the ear). Allergy can result in pressure behind the ear drum and is also a common source of ear pain. Figure 11 shows the location of major landmarks.

In the bush a simple physical examination and the additional medical history will readily (and generally accurately) distinguish the difference between an otitis media or otitis externa, and sources of pain beyond the ear. Pushing on the knob at the front of the ear (the tragus) or pulling on the ear lobe will elicit pain with an otitis externa. This will not hurt if the patient has otitis media. The history of head congestion favors otitis media.

The anatomy of the ear demonstrating the location of landmarks described in the text.

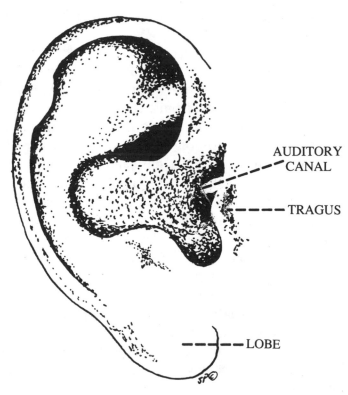

AUDITORY CANAL

TRAGUS

LOBE

Otitis Externa — Outer Ear Infection

This infection of the auditory canal is commonly called "swimmer's ear." The external auditory canal generally becomes inflamed from conditions of high humidity, accumulation of ear wax, or contact with contaminated water. Scratching the ear after itching the nose or scratching elsewhere may also be a source of this common infection.

Prevent cold air from blowing against the ear. Warm packs against the ear or instilling comfortably warm sweet oil, or even clean cooking oil, can help. Provide pain medication. Obtain professional help if the patient develops a fever, the pain becomes severe, or lymph nodes or adjacent neck tissues start swelling. Significant tissue swelling will require antibiotic treatment. Nonprescription ear drops will not clear infections, but can help with pain and local irritation.

Otitis Media — Middle Ear Infection

This condition will present in a person who has sinus congestion and possibly drainage from allergy or infection. The ear pain can be excruciating. Fever will frequently be intermittent, normal at one moment and over 103 F at other times. Fever indicates bacterial infection of the fluid trapped behind the ear drum. If the ear drum ruptures, the pain will cease immediately and the fever will drop. This drainage allows the body to cure the infection, but will result in at least temporary damage to the ear drum and decreased hearing until it heals.

Treatment will consist of providing decongestant, pain medication and oral antibiotic. An ideal decongestant is Actifed, 1 tablet 4 times daily. Give oral pain medication. The oral antibiotic is a prescription product and not a first aid item. A full description of the advanced care of ear infections will be found in *Wilderness Medicine*, to include the use of antibiotics.

Foreign Body in the Ear

These are generally of three types. Accumulation of wax plugs (cerumen), foreign objects, and living insects. Wax plugs can usually be softened with a warmed oil. This may have to be placed in the ear canal repeatedly over many days. Irrigating with room temperature water may be attempted with a bulb syringe. If a wax plugged ear becomes painful, treat as indicated in the section on otitis externa. See figure 12.

Figure 12   Bulb syringe for irrigating wounds, ear, or eye as described in the text.

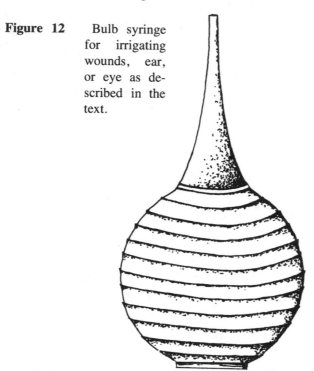

The danger in trying to remove inanimate objects is the tendency to shove them further into the ear canal or to damage the delicate ear canal lining, thus adding bleeding to your troubles. Of course, rupturing the ear drum by shoving against it would be a real unnecessary disaster. Attempt to grasp a foreign body with a pair of tweezers if you can visualize it. Do not poke blindly with anything. Irrigation may be attempted as indicated above.

A method of aiding in the management of insects in the ear canal is to drown the bug with cooking or other oil, then attempt removal. Oil seems to kill bugs quicker than water. The less struggle, the less chance for stinging, biting, or other trauma to the delicate ear canal and ear drum. Tilt the ear downward, thus hoping to slide the dead bug towards the entrance where it can be grappled. Shining a light at the ear to coax a bug out is probably futile.

Nose

Foreign Body in Nose

Foul drainage from one nostril is very suspicious of a foreign body. In adults the history of something being placed up the nose would, of course, help in the diagnosis. In a child drainage from one nostril must be considered to be a foreign body until ruled out. Have the patient try to blow his nose to remove the foreign body. With an infant it may be possible for a parent to gently puff into the baby's mouth to force the object out of the nose.

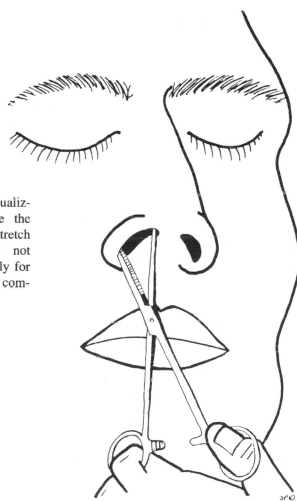

Figure 13 When visualizing inside the nose, stretch vertically, not horizontally for optimum comfort.

While having a nasal speculum would be ideal, using the emergency kit one can improvise by using the mosquito or Hartman hemostats. Spread the tips apart after placing them just inside the nostril. One can stretch the nostril without pain quite extensively, as illustrated in figure 13. Shine a light into the nostril passage and attempt to spot the foreign body. Try to grasp the object with another forceps or other instrument under direct visualization in this manner.

After removing a foreign body, be sure to check the nostril again for an additional one. Try not to push a foreign body down the back of the patient's throat where they may choke on it. If this is unavoidable, have the patient face down and bend over to decrease the chance of choking.

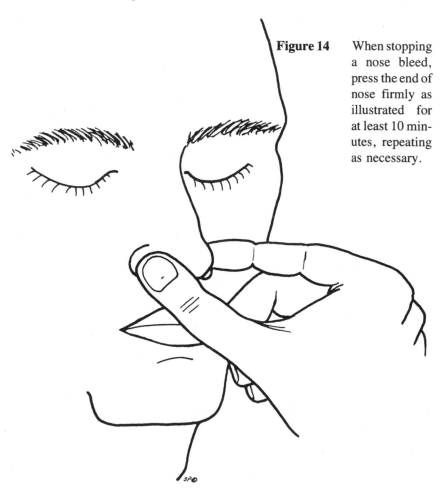

Figure 14 When stopping a nose bleed, press the end of nose firmly as illustrated for at least 10 minutes, repeating as necessary.

Nose Bleed (Epistaxis)

If nose bleeding is caused from a contusion to the nose, the bleeding is usually self limited. Bleeding that starts without trauma is generally more difficult to stop. Most bleeding is from small arteries located near the front of the nose partition, or nasal septum.

The best treatment is direct pressure. Have the victim squeeze the nose between his fingers for ten minutes by the clock (a very long time when there is no clock to watch), in the location as illustrated in figure 14. If this fails, squeeze another ten minutes. Do not blow the nose for this will dislodge clots and start the bleeding all over again.

If the bleeding is severe, have the victim sit up to prevent choking on blood and to aid in the reduction of the blood pressure in the nose. Cold compresses do little good. The field treatment of nose fractures and dislocations and advanced techniques of dealing with severe bloody noses are described in my book *Wilderness Medicine*.

Dental Pain, Lost Filling, and Trauma

Cavities may be identified by visual examination of the mouth in most cases. Dry the tooth and try to clean out any cavity found. For years oil of cloves, or eugenol, has been used to deaden dental pain. Avoid trying to apply an aspirin directly to a painful tooth, it will only make a worse mess of things. A daub of topical anesthetic such as 1% dibucaine ointment will help deaden dental pain work. Before applying the anesthetic, dry the tooth and try to clean out any cavity found. Give pain medication such as Mobigesic.

When you examine a traumatized mouth and find a tooth that is rotated, or dislocated in any direction, do not push the tooth back into place. Further movement may disrupt the tooth's blood and nerve supply. If the tooth is at all secure leave it alone. The musculature of the lips and tongue will generally gently push the tooth back into place and keep it there.

A fractured tooth with exposed pink substance that is bleeding, is showing exposed nerve. This tooth will need protection with eugenol as indicated above. This is actually a dental emergency that should be treated by a dentist immediately.

If a tooth is knocked out, replace it into the socket immediately. If this cannot be done, have the victim hold the tooth under their

tongue or in their lower lip until it can be implanted. In any case
time is a matter of great importance. A tooth left out too long will
be rejected by the body as a foreign substance.

All of the above problems will mean that a soft diet and
avoidance of chewing with the affected tooth for many days will
be necessary. Trauma that can cause any of the above may also
result in fractures of the tooth below the gum line and of the alveolar
ridge affecting several teeth, note figure 15. Persons suffering dental
trauma should be taken to a dentist as soon as possible.

Figure 15   Possible dental fracture, or break, lines.

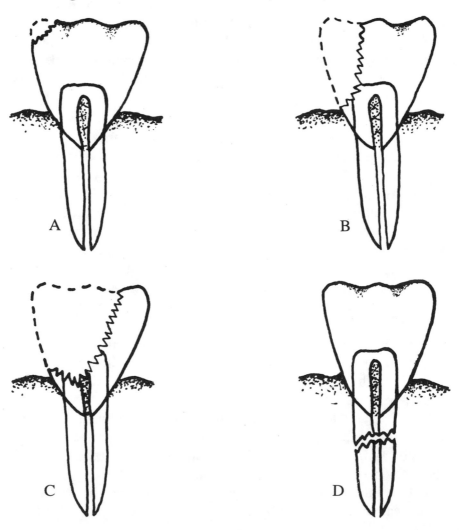

3. ABDOMINAL PAIN AND OTHER PROBLEMS

Any abdominal pain that lasts longer than 1 hour is cause for serious concern — seek help if possible. Possible clues to the cause of abdominal pain are indicated in Table 1, below.

TABLE 1
Symptoms and Signs of Abdominal Pathology

	Burning	Nausea	Food Related	Diarrhea	Fever
Gastritis/ulcer	xx	x	xx		
Pancreatitis	xx	x	x		x
Hiatal Hernia	xx		x		
Gall Bladder		xx	xx		(x)
Appendicitis		x			x
Gastro-enteritis		xx		xx	x
Diverticulitis				xx	x
Hepatitis		xx	x		x
Food Poisoning		xx	xx	xx	x

Diagnosis is frequently derived by the type of pain, location, cause, fever — all from the history — as well as certain aspects of the physical exam and the clinical course that develops.

The possibility of **APPENDICITIS** is a major concern as it can occur in any age group, and that includes healthy wilderness travelers. It is fortunately uncommon. The classic presentation of this illness is a vague feeling of discomfort around the umbilicus (navel). Temperature may be low grade, 99.6 to 100.6 at first. Within a matter of hours the discomfort turns to pain and localizes in the right lower quadrant, most frequently on a point 1/3 of the way between the navel and the very top of the right pelvic bone (anterior-superior iliac spine), as illustrated in figure 16. This pain syndrome can be elicited from the patient by asking two questions: Where did you first start hurting? (belly button); Now where do you hurt? (right lower quadrant as described). Those answers mean appendicitis until it is ruled out.

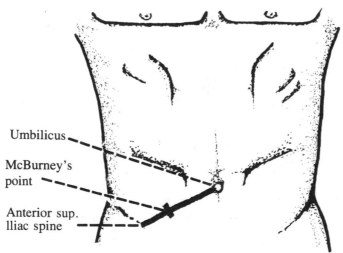

Figure 16   The location of McBurney's Point, the location of maximum pain in classic appendicitis.

Nausea and Vomiting

Nausea and vomiting are frequently caused by infections known as gastroenteritis. Many times these are viral so that antibiotics are of no value. These infections will usually resolve without treatment in 24 to 48 hours. Fever seldom is high, but may briefly be high in some cases. Fever should not persist above 100 degrees longer than 12 hours. Treatment may be with meclizine from the medical kit. Professional help should be sought if fever persists longer than 24 hours, or if severe pain is also present.

Motion Sickness

To prevent and treat motion sickness, a very useful non-Rx drug is meclizine 25 mg, taken 1 hour prior to departure for all day protection. There is minimal drowsiness or other side effects with this medication. Transderm Scōp, a patch containing scopalamine, has been developed for prevention of motion sickness, but this requires an Rx. Each patch may be worn behind the ear for 3 days as shown in figure 17. It is fairly expensive, but very worth while if you are prone to this malady. There tends to be a higher frequency of side effects with this medication in elderly people, such as visual problems, confusion, and loss of temperature regulation.

Figure 17   The point of application for the Transderm Scōp patch, used to prevent motion sickness.

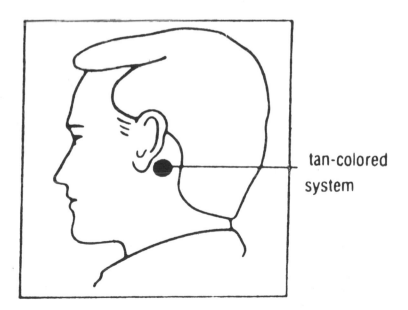

tan-colored system

Diarrhea

Diarrhea is the expulsion of watery stool. This malady is usually self limited, but can be a threat to life, depending upon its cause and extent. Diarrhea can be a symptom of diverticulitis, cholera, food or water contamination, parasites such as *Giardia lamblia*, colitis and other inflammations of the bowel, and rarely with appendicitis and gall bladder disease.

Giardia lamblia is a parasite which causes concern in outdoors travelers as it is frequently diagnosed as a cause of diarrhea in backpackers, canoeists and campers in the United States. This parasite is also spread by beaver populations. It is probably being over-diagnosed considerably. Most stools from diarrhea victims continue to show other causes such as *E. coli* and rotovirus infections which, let's face it folks, we did not catch from a beaver but from a fellow human being. *Giardia* has an incubation period of about 7-21 days usually, so most victims should not become ill until after they return home. Treatment is with specific antibiotics.

The first aid treatment for diarrhea is the use of Diasorb from the medical kit or Pepto-Bismol. Adequate fluid replacement should be encouraged, even though the person feels like the fluid is just running right through them. Avoid dehydration!

4. SPRAINS, FRACTURES, AND DISLOCATIONS

Acute Joint Injury

Proper care of joint injuries must be started immediately. Rest, Ice, Compression, and Elevation (RICE) form the basis of good first aid management. Cold should be applied for the first 2 days, as continuously as possible. Afterward, applying heat for 20 minutes, 4 times daily is helpful. Cold decreases the circulation, which lessens bleeding and swelling. Heat increases the circulation, which then aids the healing process. This technique applies to all injuries including muscle contusions and bruises.

Elevate the involved joint, if possible. Wrap with elastic bandage or cloth tape to immobilize the joint and provide moderate support once walking or use of the joint begins. Take care that the wrappings are not so tightly applied that they cut off the circulation.

Use crutches or other support to take enough weight off an injured ankle and knee to the point that increased pain is not experienced. The patient should not use an injured joint if use causes pain, as this indicates further strain on the already stressed ligaments or fracture. Conversely, if use of the injured part does not cause pain, additional damage is not being done even if there is considerable swelling.

If the victim must walk on an injured ankle or knee, and doing so causes considerable pain, then support it the best way possible (wrapping, crutches, decreased carrying load, tight boot for ankle injury) and realize that further damage is being done, but that in your opinion the situation warrants such a sacrifice. Under emergency movement conditions; a boot should not be removed from an injured ankle as it may be impossible to replace it. However, one must avoid too much compression of the soft tissue swelling to prevent circulation impairment.

Wrapping an ankle with an ace bandage is easy. The so-called figure eight technique is illustrated in figure 18. Simply wrap around the ankle, under and around the foot and layer as shown.

Wrapping a knee is similarly performed using a figure eight technique, as shown in figure 19. These wraps provide compression and slight support. They should never be applied so tight that they cause discomfort or cut off circulation.

Pain medications may be given as needed, but elevation and decreased use will provide considerable pain relief.

Figure 18   Example of properly wrapped support dress- of figure eight technique around an ankle.

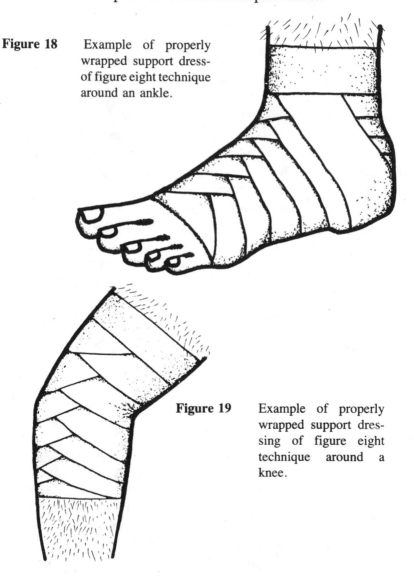

Figure 19   Example of properly wrapped support dres- sing of figure eight technique around a knee.

Dislocations

If the joint in question is deformed and/or the patient cannot move it, then the joint has suffered either a severe sprain or dislocation. Support the joint with sling or splinting in such a manner that further stress is not applied to the joint.

For the field treatment of specific dislocations, please refer to my book *Wilderness Medicine*. These techniques are beyond the scope of first aid, but if you plan a trip significantly away from medical help, replacement of shoulder, elbow, finger, and nose dislocations can reduce pain and facilitate long evacuations.

Fractures

Fracture is the medical term for a broken bone. Fractures have several critical aspects to consider during management: 1) loss of circulation or nerve damage if bone spicules press against these structures due to deformity of the fracture; 2) introduction of infection if the skin is broken at or near the fracture site; 3) failure of the bone to mend properly due to improper alignment of bone fragments.

At times it will be uncertain whether or not a fracture actually exists. There will be point tenderness, frequently swelling and discoloration over the fracture site or the generalized area, and in obvious cases, deformity and loss of stability. If doubt exists, splint and treat for pain, avoiding the use of the involved part. Within a few days the pain will have diminished and the crises may be over. If not, the suspicion of fracture will loom even larger.

People frequently will say *"Well, I can move it, it must not be broken!"* This is not true. The pain associated with movement may discourage movement, but it certainly does not prevent it.

With proper splinting the pain involved with a fracture will decrease dramatically. Pain medication should be provided as soon as possible. A proper splint is well padded to protect underlying skin from developing pressure sores. It should also immobilize the joint above and below the fracture site. Fracture splinting requires common sense — and sometimes imagination when fabricating some first aid device from available items such as ski poles, backpack frame parts, tree branches — even boots, eye glass frames, and articles of clothing.

Reduction, or correction, of fractures should be left to the hands of skilled persons. The adage "splint them as they lie" is the golden rule in handling fractures. However, if obvious circulation damage is occurring, namely the pulses beyond the fracture site have ceased, the extremity is turning blue and cold to the touch, or numbness is apparent in the portion of the limb beyond the fracture, angulations of the fracture should be straightened to attempt to eliminate the pressure damage. Broken bone edges can be very sharp — in fact a laceration of the blood vessels and nerves may have already occurred, thus causing the above symptoms. An attempt at correcting alignment may cause further damage, thus the aforementioned adage "splint them as they lie."

5. BITES AND STINGS

Animal Bites

Animal bite wounds must be vigorously cleaned. The wound should generally be covered with triple antibiotic ointment and a pressure dressing. The patient should be seen by a physician as soon as possible. Tetanus immunization must be current within 5 years.

Rabies

Rabies can be transmitted on the North American continent by several species of mammals, namely skunk, bat, fox, coyote, raccoon, bobcat, and wolf. Hawaii is the only rabies free state. Dogs and cats in the United States have a low incidence of rabies. Information from local departments of health will indicate if rabies is currently of concern in these animals.

The incubation period in a human is 1 to 2 months. Rabies is a vicious disease that is usually fatal once it clinically develops. Because of this, there is generous use of rabies vaccine and immune globulin. Although there have been only 9 cases of rabies reported between 1980 and 1987 in the United States, approximately 20,000 people are vaccinated here yearly to prevent this disease.

Treatment of Insect Bites and Stings

Honey bee — also wasp, yellow jackets, and hornets are members of the order *Hymenoptera*. Stings from these insects hurt instantly and the pain lingers. The danger comes from the fact that some persons are "hypersensitive" to the venom and can have an immediate *anaphylactic shock* which is life-threatening. Fire ants and other insects may also cause an anaphylactic reaction.

The pain of stings and local skin reactions to bites can be alleviated by almost anything applied topically. Best choices are cold packs, dibucaine ointment from the medical kit, or a piece of Spenco 2nd Skin and the use of oral pain medication such as Mobigesic. Swelling can be prevented and/or treated with oral antihistamine such as the Benadryl 25 mg taken 4 times daily.

The puss caterpillar (*Megalopyge opercularis*) of the southern US and the gypsy moth caterpillar (*Lymantria dispar*) of the northeastern US have bristles that cause an almost immediate skin rash and welt formation. Treatment includes patting the victim with a piece of adhesive tape to remove these bristles. Thoroughly cleanse the area with soap and water. A patch of Spenco 2nd Skin is very cooling. Give Benadryl 25 mg, one capsule 4 times daily.

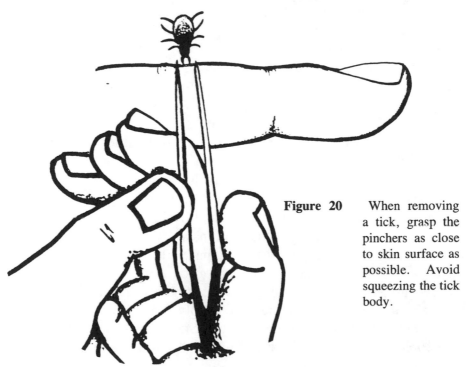

Figure 20   When removing a tick, grasp the pinchers as close to skin surface as possible. Avoid squeezing the tick body.

Tick bites are of increased concern due to the diseases that can be transmitted by these little fellows. Lyme disease, Rocky Mountain spotted fever, Colorado tick fever, and tick paralysis are amongst these diseases. Remove the tick by grasping the victim's skin with the splinter forceps (tweezers) just where the tick has bitten the victim as illustrated in figure 20. Remove by pulling straight up, probably also taking a small piece of skin as the tick pincers hang on tightly. I have not found heating the tick with a hot paper clip, using alcohol, finger nail polish remover, or other chemical means very successful.

Anaphylactic Shock

While most commonly due to insect stings, this severe form of life-threatening shock may be encountered as a serious allergic reaction to medications, shell fish and other foods, or anything to which one has become profoundly allergic. Those developing anaphylaxis generally have warnings of their severe sensitivity in the form of welts (urticaria) forming all over their body immediately after exposure, the development of an asthmatic attack with respiratory wheezing, or the onset of symptoms of shock. After an exposure with such severe warning symptoms, the concern is that the next exposure might produce increased symptoms or even the shock state known as anaphylaxis.

This deadly form of shock can begin within seconds of exposure. It cannot be treated as shock would normally be handled, with elevation of the feet above heart level. The only life-saving remedy is to administer the drug called epinephrine (Adrenalin). It is available for emergency use as a component of a prepackaged prescription kit called the "Anakit" or in a special automatic injectable syringe called the EpiPen. Note illustrations of each type of kit in figure 21.

The Anakit is recommended as it contains two injections of epinephrine, rather than one and the cost is about half that of the EpiPen. Normal dosage is .3 cc for an adult of the 1:1000 epinephrine solution given "subQ" (in the fatty layer beneath the skin). This may have to be repeated in 15 to 20 minutes if the symptoms of wheezing or shock start to return. The Anakit contains a chewable antihistamine which should also be taken immediately, but antihistamines are of no value in treating the shock or asthmatic component of anaphylaxis.

Anyone experiencing anaphylactic reactions should be evacuated to medical care, even though they have responded to the epinephrine. They are at risk of the condition returning and they should be monitored carefully over the next 24 hours.

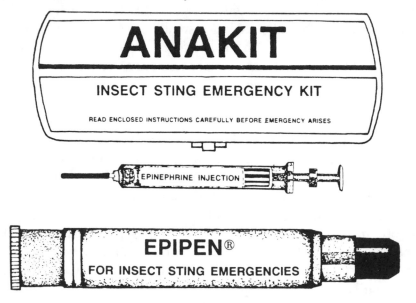

Figure 21   The "Anakit" and "EpiPen" used to treat severe insect reactions.

Poisonous Snake Bite

Not everyone bitten by a poisonous snake will have envenomation injury — fully 20% of rattlesnake and 30% of cotton mouth water moccasin and copperhead bites will not envenomate during their bite. DO NOT APPLY COLD — this is associated with increased tissue damage. 1) Immobilize the injured part at heart level or slightly above in a position of function. 2) Apply an elastic bandage with a firm wrap from the bite site towards the body, leaving the bite exposed if you have an Extractor for further treatment, covered if you do not. 3) Apply suction with the Extractor. Making incisions actually decreases the amount of venom that can be removed with this device. If applied within 3 minutes as much as 35% of the venom may be removed with the Extractor. After 1/2 hour, less than 3% more will be removed, so further suction can be terminated. 4) Treat for shock and evacuate to professional medical help.

The Extractor, figure 22, has simplified the field care of snake bite due to its high amount of vacuum and effectiveness. It must be carried by anyone entering an area with poisonous snakes.

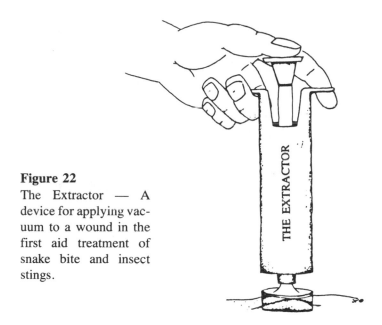

Figure 22
The Extractor — A device for applying vacuum to a wound in the first aid treatment of snake bite and insect stings.

Black Widow Spider Bite

The black widow spider is generally glossy black with a red hourglass mark on the abdomen, figure 23. Sometimes the hourglass mark is merely a red dot or the two parts of the hourglass do not connect. At times the coat is not shiny and it may contain white. The bite may be only a pin-prick, but generally a dull cramping pain begins within one quarter of an hour and this may spread gradually until it involves the entire body. The muscles may go into spasms and the abdomen become board-like. The pain can be excruciating. Nausea, vomiting, swelling of eyelids, weakness, anxiety (naturally), and pain on breathing may all develop. A healthy adult usually survives, with the pain abating in several hours and the remaining symptoms disappearing in several days.

An ice cube on the bite, if available, may reduce local pain. A specific antivenin is available which should be given by a physician to persons under 16 and over 65, heart or kidney patients, or those with very severe symptoms. Pain relief can be sought by using the Mobigesic or other pain medication.

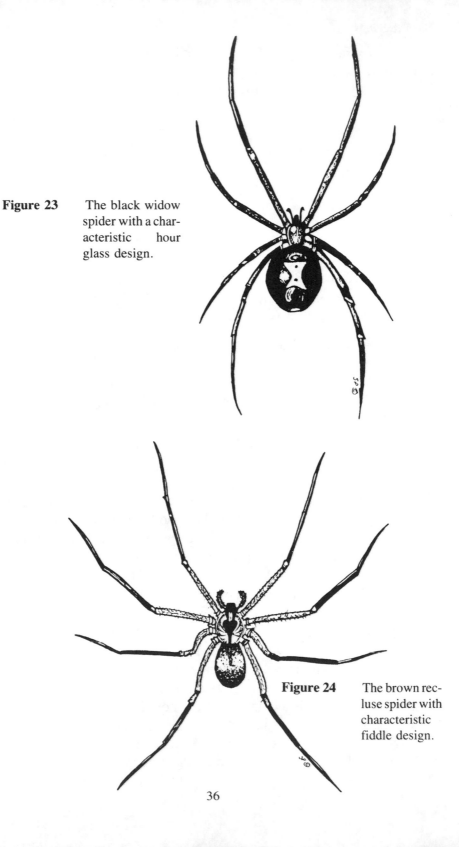

Figure 23 The black widow spider with a characteristic hour glass design.

Figure 24 The brown recluse spider with characteristic fiddle design.

Brown Recluse Spider

A brown coat with a black violin marking on the cephalothorax, or top part of the spider, distinguishes this spider, figure 24. The initial bite is mild and may be overlooked at the time. In an hour or two a slight redness may appear and by several hours a small blister appears at the bite site. At times the wound begins to look like a bull's eye with several rings of red and blanched circles around the bite. The blister ruptures, forming a crust, which then sloughs off. A large necrotic ulcer forms which gradually enlarges. Over the first 36 hours, vomiting, fever, skin rash and joint pain may develop. In severe cases the red blood cells break down in the circulation.

Apply ice to the wound as soon as possible. An antivenin has been developed from rabbits and is being used experimentally. Avoid the application of heat to this wound, even though it is inflamed and necrotic. Apply triple antibiotic ointment from the topical bandaging unit and cover with Spenco 2nd Skin dressing. Specific medical treatment is available and these victims should be evacuated to professional medical help as soon as possible.

Scorpion Sting

Most North American scorpion stings are relatively harmless. Stings usually cause only localized pain and slight swelling. The wound may feel numb. Benadryl and Mobigesic may be all that is required for treatment. A cold pack will help relieve local pain.

The potentially lethal *Centruroides sculptuatus* is the exception to this rule. This yellow colored scorpion lives in Mexico, New Mexico, Arizona, and the California side of the Colorado River. The sting causes immediate, severe pain with swelling and subsequent numbness. The neurotoxin injected with this bite may cause respiratory failure. Respiratory assistance may be required (see Appendix B). Tapping on the wound lightly with your finger will cause the patient to withdraw due to severe pain. This is an unusual reaction and does not occur with most insect stings. A specific antivenin is available in Mexico and is also produced by the Poisonous Animals Laboratory at Arizona State University for local use. In addition to the antivenin, other medications can be administered by a physician to combat the ill effects of the bite. Provide pain medication and treat for shock as necessary. These patients should be seen by a physician as soon as possible.

6. COLD AND HEAT INJURIES

Hypothermia

The term "hypothermia" refers to the lowering of the body's core temperature to 95° F (35° C); "profound hypothermia" is a core temperature lower than 90° F (32° C). Another important point is that the term "hypothermia" applies to two distinctly different diseases. One is "chronic hypothermia," the slow onset hypothermia of the outdoors traveler exposed to conditions too cold for their equipment to adequately protect them; the other is "acute," or "immersion hypothermia," the rapid onset hypothermia of a person immersed in cold water.

Hypothermia is the most likely of the environmental injuries that will be encountered in the outdoors. Prevention is the hallmark of survival, in fact hypothermia has been called the killer of the unprepared. It is most important to attempt to prevent hypothermia.

The factors that protect trip members include:

1. PROPER PRE-TRIP PHYSICAL CONDITIONING
2. ADEQUATE NUTRITION
3. PREVENTION OF PHYSICAL EXHAUSTION
4. PREVENTION OF DEHYDRATION
5. ADEQUATE CLOTHING
6. REPLACEMENT CLOTHING

Chronic Hypothermia

The essential ingredients in surviving this situation are: being prepared to prevent it, recognizing it if it occurs, and knowing how to treat it. Dampness and wind are the most devastating factors to be considered. Dampness as it can reduce the insulation of clothing and cause evaporative heat loss. Wind as the increased convection heat loss can readily strip away body energy, the so called "wind chill" effect, figure 25. Remember, it is possible to die of hypothermia in temperatures far above freezing — in fact most hypothermia deaths occur in the 30° to 50° F (-1° to 10°C) range.

Detection of hypothermia is generally made by two observations. The first is to watch for exhaustion. An exhausted person is not necessarily hypothermic, yet. But he will be unless he can obtain adequate rest and have adequate clothing to protect him from heat loss during rest.

The second is loss of coordination. A person who cannot walk a straight 30 foot (9 meter) line is hypothermic. This same test was formerly used by the police to detect inebriation, which also causes loss of coordination. Both impair mental function. For that reason, when hypothermia is detected in a person, their judgement must be suspect. More than not trusting their decisions, these people actually need help. They must be treated for hypothermia.

The treatment for hypothermia is basically:

1.   Prevent further heat loss. Wet clothing must be removed and replaced with dry clothing. At the very least, it must be covered with a rain jacket and pants — and this in turn covered with more insulation.

2.   Treat dehydration. Hypothermia causes vasoconstriction

which in effect shrinks the fluid volume of the victim. This is only one reason for dehydration, but all hypothermic people are, indeed, very dehydrated. This volume needs replacement.

3.   Treat the victim gently. A very cold person can suffer cardiac rhythm problems if they are jarred around. If they are being carried during an evacuation, avoid bumping them along the ground or dropping them from a stretcher.

4.   Add heat. If the patient can stand, and you can build a fire, do it! And have them stand comfortably near it. A roaring fire can replace a massive number of calories and practically speaking, if a patient can stand on their own by the fire, they are not so profoundly hypothermic that you would have to worry about rewarming shock.

5.   Avoid rewarming shock. Persons who are unable to stand are so ill that if they were reheated too rapidly, they could be adversely affected. The dehydration of hypothermia causes a sub-stantial decrease in their fluid volume. So much so that a sudden rewarming can result in shock, even death. Note: this is a concern of the chronic hypothermic, not the acute (immersion) hypothermic victim.

6.   Understand afterdrop. As victims were being reheated it was noted that their core temperature continued to drop before starting to rise. This is called "afterdrop." It was originally thought to be a cause of death, but the significant reason for death in the chronic hypothermic is actually rewarming shock. All persons will have afterdrop, which is related to the rate of cooling that was taking place before the rewarming process started. It amounts to an equilibration phenomenon. Afterdrop is a serious problem in the treatment of acute (immersion) hypothermia, but is probably not of much concern in the chronic hypothermic. The amount of drop can be decreased by adding sufficient heat so that the equilibration process is minimized at the core.

7.   Avoid adding cold. Never rub the person with snow or allow further exposure to the cold. It is probably best to avoid undressing the person exposed to the environment — do this in a sleeping bag or other sheltered area if at all possible. Try to warm water before giving the patient, if possible.

8.   Allow rest. These patients are at or near exhaustion. Rest is mandatory to replace the high energy compounds that are required

to shiver, work, and otherwise generate heat. If the resting person is being adequately insulated from further heat loss, there is no reason why they cannot be allowed to sleep. It is therapeutic. Do not shake or slap a hypothermic individual (see item 3 above).

Deepening hypothermia will lead to a semi-comatose state and worse. This victim needs to be evacuated to help. Wrap to prevent further heat loss and transport. Chemical heat packs, etc., can be added to the wrap to help offset further heat loss, but care must be taken not to burn the victim. If evacuation is not feasible, heat will have to be added slowly to avoid re-warming shock. Huddling with two rescuers naked with the victim in an adequate sleeping bag may be the only alternative. During cold weather trips it is best to insure that two trip members are carrying semi-rectangular bags that can twin, thus providing a means of adequately huddling 3 persons in a bag. Mummy bags are too small to implement this technique, although they make the ideal winter bag for personal use.

Acute Hypothermia

Acute hypothermia is the term applied to hypothermia which occurs in less than 2 hours. This generally means cold water immersion. If the air temperature and the water temperature add to less than 100° F (38° C), there is a risk of acute hypothermia if a person falls into the water. As a rule of thumb, a person who has been in water of 50° F (10° C) or less for a period of 20 minutes or longer, is suffering from a severe amount of heat loss. That individual's thermal mass has been so reduced that they are in a potentially serious condition. They should not be allowed to move around as this will increase the blood flow to their very cold skin and facilitate a profound circulatory induced afterdrop; one that is so great as to be potentially lethal. If this same person is simply wrapped as a litter case and not provided outside heat, there is a real danger of them cooling below a lethal level due to this profound amount of heat loss.

The ideal treatment is rapid re-warming of the acute hypothermic by placing them in hot water (110° F, or 43° C) to allow rapid replacement of heat. These people may have an almost normal core temperature initially, but one that is destined to drop dramatically as their body equilibrates the heat store from their core to their very cold mantle. A roaring fire can be a life saver. If not available, huddling two naked rescuers with the victim in a large sleeping bag may be the only answer — the same therapy that might have to be employed in the field treatment of chronic hypothermia under some conditions.

SIGNS AND SYMPTOMS OF HYPOTHERMIA

CORE TEMP.	SIGNS AND SYMPTOMS
99° to 97°F (37° to 36°C)	Normal temperature range Shivering may begin
97° to 95°F (36° to 35°C)	Cold sensation, goose bumps, unable to perform complex tasks with hands, shivering can be mild to severe, skin numb
95° to 93°F (35° to 34°C)	Shivering intense, muscle incoordination becomes apparent, movements slow and labored, stumbling pace, mild confusion, may appear alert, unable to walk 30 ft. line properly — BEST FIELD TEST FOR EARLY HYPOTHERMIA
93° to 90°F (34° to 32°C)	Violent shivering persists, difficulty speaking, sluggish thinking, amnesia starts to appear and may be retrograde, gross muscle movements sluggish, unable to use hands, stumbles frequently, difficulty speaking, signs of depression
90° to 86°F 32° to 30°C)	Shivering stops in chronic hypothermia, exposed skin blue or puffy, muscle coordination very poor with inability to walk, confusion, incoherent, irrational behavior, BUT MAY BE ABLE TO MAINTAIN POSTURE AND THE APPEARANCE OF PSYCHOLOGICAL CONTACT
86° to 82°F (30° to 27.7°C)	Muscles severely rigid, semiconscious, stupor, loss of psychological contact, pulse and respirations slow, pupils can dilate
82° to 78°F (27 to 25.5°C)	Unconsciousness, heart beat and respiration erratic, pulse and heart beat may be inapparent, muscle tendon reflexes cease
78° to 75°F (25° to 24°C)	Pulmonary edema, failure of cardiac and respiratory centers, probable death, DEATH MAY OCCUR BEFORE THIS LEVEL
64°F (17.7°C)	Lowest recorded temperature of chronic hypothermia survivor, Chicago 1951
48.2°F (9°C)	Lowest recorded temperature of induced hypothermia in surgical patient with survival, 1958

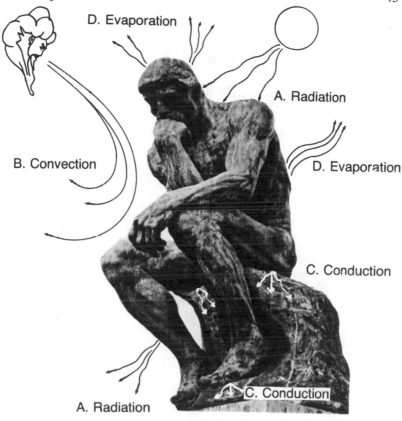

Figure 25   An illustration of the physical modes of heat transfer.

The mechanisms of heat transfer between man and the environment include: A. *Radiation* - heat transferred by electromagnetic waves from warm to cooler objects; B. *Convection* - heat transfer by molecules of air or fluid moving between areas of unequal temperature; C. *Conduction* - heat exchange between objects in contact; D. *Evaporation* - heat loss by water molecules diffusing from the body surface, by sweating, and by environmental wetting when this water changes from a liquid to a vapor state. The above methods are further explained in the text.

Frostbite

Frostbite is the freezing of tissue. Surface skin goes through several phases before this occurs. The freezing process requires predisposing risk factors to be present before the events leading to frostbite are initiated. Outside temperatures must be below freezing for frostbite to occur, in fact skin temperature must be cooled to between 22° to 24° F (-5.5° C to -4.4° C) before tissue will freeze. The underlying physical condition of the victim, length of cold

FAHRENHEIT WIND CHILL EQUIVALENT TEMPERATURE

Wind Speed MPH	TEMPERATURE FAHRENHEIT																					
Calm	50	40	35	30	25	20	15	10	5	0	-5	-10	-15	-20	-25	-30	-35	-40	-45	-50	-55	-60
5	48	37	33	27	21	16	12	6	1	-5	-11	-15	-20	-26	-31	-36	-41	-47	-52	-57	-65	-70
10	40	28	21	16	9	4	-2	-9	-15	-24	-27	-33	-38	-46	-52	-58	-64	-70	-75	-83	-90	-95
15	36	22	16	9	1	-5	-11	-18	-25	-32	-40	-45	-51	-58	-65	-72	-77	-85	-90	-99	-105	-110
20	32	18	12	4	-4	-10	-17	-25	-32	-39	-46	-53	-60	-67	-75	-82	-89	-96	-102	-110	-115	-120
25	30	16	7	0	-7	-15	-22	-29	-37	-44	-52	-59	-67	-74	-83	-88	-96	-104	-111	-118	-125	-135
30	28	13	5	-2	-11	-18	-26	-33	-41	-48	-56	-63	-70	-79	-87	-94	-101	-109	-115	-125	-130	-140
35	27	11	3	-4	-13	-20	-27	-35	-43	-51	-60	-67	-72	-82	-90	-98	-105	-113	-120	-129	-135	-146
40	26	10	1	-6	-15	-21	-29	-37	-45	-53	-62	-69	-76	-85	-94	-100	-107	-115	-125	-132	-140	-150

Exposed Flesh Can Freeze in 60 Seconds

Exposed Flesh Can Freeze in 30 Seconds

"WIND CHILL CHART - FAHRENHEIT"

NOTE 1.   The above chart has been based upon the Siple Equation and reflects Wind Chill Equivalent temperatures in Fahrenheit.

NOTE 2.   At low wind speeds, relative humidity and radiant heat are more important than wind speed in determining equivalent temperature comfort.

NOTE 3.   Most charts indicate that at wind speeds over 40 mph there is little additional wind chill effect. This is a reflection of an error in the basic equation at these higher wind speeds and is not correct. Heat loss IS magnified by these higher wind speeds, but the chart is an accurate indicator of equivalent temperature at speeds lower than 40 mph.

contact, and type of cold contact (such as cold metal or fuel) are other important factors leading to frostbite.

Traditionally, several degrees of frostbite are recognized, but the treatment for all is the same and the actual degree of severity will not be known until after the patient has been treated and the amount of damage then readily identified. Deeply frostbitten flesh will not indent when pressed upon, while superficial injury will also be waxy colored and cold, but will indent.

When superficial frostbite is suspected, thaw immediately so that it does not become a more serious, deep frostbite. Warm the hands by withdrawing them into the parka through the sleeves — avoid opening the front of the parka to minimize heat loss. Feet should be thawed against a companion or cupped in your own hands in a roomy sleeping bag, or otherwise in an insulated environment. NEVER, NEVER rub snow on a frostbitten area.

For victims with deep frostbite, rapid rewarming in 110° F (43° C) water is the most effective treatment. This thawing may take 20 to 30 minutes, but it should be continued until all paleness of the tips of the fingers or toes has turned pink or burgundy red, but no longer. This will be very painful and will require pain medication. Refreezing would result in substantial tissue loss. The frozen part should not be thawed if there is any possibility of refreezing the part. Also, once the victim has been thawed, very careful management of the thawed part is required. The patient will become a stretcher case if the foot is involved. For that reason, it may be necessary to leave the foot or leg(s) frozen and allow the victim to walk back to the evacuation point. Tissue damage increases with the length of time that it is allowed to remain frozen, but this damage is less than the refreezing destruction.

Immersion Foot

It is essential that anyone going into the outdoors know how to prevent this injury. It results from wet, cool conditions with temperature exposures from 68° F (20° C) down to freezing. To prevent this problem avoid non-breathing (rubber) footwear when possible, dry the feet and change wool or polypro socks when feet become wet or sweaty (every 3 to 4 hours, if necessary), and periodically elevate, air, dry, and massage the feet to promote circulation. Avoid tight, constrictive clothing. At night footwear must absolutely be removed and socks changed to dry ones, or simply removed and feet dried before retiring to the sleeping bag.

There are two clinical stages of immersion foot. In the initial stage the foot is cold, swollen, waxy, mottled with dark burgundy to blue splotches. This foot is spongy to touch, whereas the frozen foot is very hard. Skin is sodden and friable. Loss of feeling makes walking difficult. The second stage lasts from days to weeks. The feet are swollen, red and hot. Blisters form and infection and gangrene are common problems. The pain from immersion foot can be life-long and massive tissue injury can easily develop.

Treatment would include providing the victim 10 grains of aspirin every 6 hours to help decrease platelet adhesion and promote blood circulaton. This injury is the only wilderness situation in which alcohol plays a proper role. Providing 1 ounce of hard liquor every hour while awake and 2 ounces every 2 hours during sleeping hours, helps dilate blood vessels and increase the flow of blood to the feet. Immediate stretcher evacuation is necessary.

Other cold injuries such as chilblains, frozen lung, etc., are less threatening and will not seriously injure trip participants. A full treatment of the prevention, diagnosis, and treatment of cold injuries is covered in my book *Hypothermia: Death by Exposure*. Additional material on these subjects can be obtained from several of the books in the reference section.

Heat Cramps

Salt depletion can result in nausea, twitching of muscle groups and at times severe cramping of abdominal muscles, legs, or elsewhere. Treatment consists of stretching the muscles involved (avoid overly aggressive massage), resting in a cool environment, and replacing salt losses. Generally 10 to 15 grams (1/3 to 1/2 oz) of salt and generous water replacement should be adequate treatment.

Heat Exhaustion

This is a classic example of SHOCK, but in this case encountered while working in a hot environment and due to a heat stress injury. The body has dilated the blood vessels in the skin, attempting to divert heat from the core to the surface for cooling. However, this dilation is so pronounced, coupled with the profuse sweating and loss of fluid — also a part of the cooling process, that the blood pressure to the entire system falls too low to adequately supply the brain and the other organs. The patient will have a rapid heart rate, and will have the other findings associated with shock: pale color, nausea, dizziness, headache, and a light-headed feeling. Generally the patient is sweating profusely, but this may not be the case. Skin temperature may be low, normal, or mildly elevated.

Treat as for shock. Have the patient lie down immediately, and elevate the feet to increase the blood supply to the head. Also, provide copious water; 10 to 15 grams of salt would also be helpful, but water is the most important. Give a minimum of 1 to 2 quarts. Obviously, fluids can only be administered if the patient is conscious. If unconscious, elevate the feet 3 feet above head level and try to protect from the potential of accidentally inhaling vomit. Try to revive with stimulation, such as contact with the person. Give water when the patient awakens.

Heat Stroke

Heat stroke, or sun stroke as it is also called, represents the complete breakdown of the heat control process (thermal regulation). Core temperatures rise over 105° F (40.5° C) rapidly and will soon exceed 115° F (46° C) and result in death if this condition is not treated aggressively. THIS IS A TRUE MEDICAL EMERGENCY. The patient will be confused and rapidly become unconscious.

Immediately move the victim into shade or erect a hasty barrier for shade. If possible employ immediate immersion in ice water to lower the temperature. Once the core temperature lowers to 102° F the victim is removed and the temperature carefully monitored. It may continue to fall or suddenly rise again.

Further cooling with wet cloths may suffice. IV solutions of normal saline are started in the clinic setting — in the wilderness, douse the victim with the coolest water possible. Massage limbs to allow the cooler blood of the extremities to return to core circulation more readily. Sacrifice your water supply — if necessary, fan and massage to provide the best coolant effect possible. This person should be evacuated as soon as possible, for his thermal regulation mechanism is quite unstable and will be labile for an unknown length of time. He should be placed under a physician's care as soon as possible.

Prickly Heat

This is a heat rash caused by the entrapment of sweat in glands in the skin. This can result in irritation and frequently severe itching. Treatment includes cooling and drying the involved area and avoiding conditions that may induce sweating for awhile. Topical medications are less effective than the steps just mentioned.

APPENDIX A

Cardio-Pulmonary Resuscitation

RESCUE BREATHING — New techniques for rescue breathing were established in 1986. The best way to provide artificial respiration is by using the mouth-to-mouth technique. The victim should be shaken by the shoulder to make sure that he is unconscious. If the victim is not lying flat on his back, roll him over, moving the entire body at one time as a total unit. The rescuer should place his face near the victim's to ascertain whether or not air movement is occurring through the mouth or nose. If breathing is absent,the throat and mouth should be cleared of foreign material (snow, mucus, dental plates, vomit, etc.) by inserting the fingers into the mouth and scooping this material out.

To open the victim's airway, use the head-tilt/chin-lift method, rather than the head-tilt/neck-lift method as taught before 1986. Place one hand on the victim's forehead and apply firm, backwards pressure with the palm to tilt the head back. Also place the fingers of the other hand under the bony part of the lower jaw near the chin and lift to bring the chin forward and the teeth almost shut, thus supporting the jaw and helping to tilt the head back, as indicated in figure 26. In case of suspected neck injury, use the chin-lift without the head-tilt technique. The nose is pinched shut by using the thumb and index finger of the hand on the forehead.

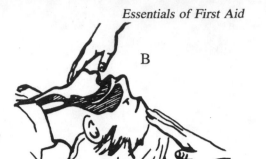

Figure 26   The head tilt/chin lift method of opening the airway in an unconscious person.

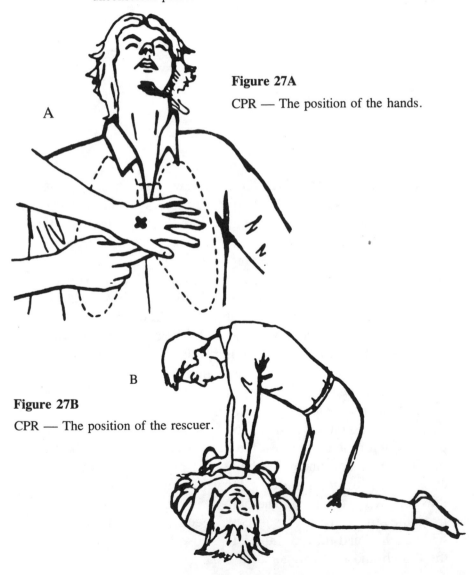

Figure 27A

CPR — The position of the hands.

Figure 27B

CPR — The position of the rescuer.

The chin-lift method will place tension on the tongue and throat structures to insure that the air passage will open. This opening of the air passage may be all that is required to allow the victim to start breathing again. Reassess breathing again by looking for the chest raising or falling, listening for air escaping during expiration, and feeling the movement of air.

Give two initial breaths of 1 to 1½ seconds each, as opposed to the "4 quick breaths" previously recommended. The rescuer should take a breath after each ventilation. If the initial attempt to ventilate does not work, reposition the victim's head and try again. If ventilation still does not work, proceed with foreign-body airway obstruction maneuvers. (See page 53.) If it does work, assess circulatory status and provide cardiac compressions if necessary. If pulses can be felt, but the patient is not breathing on their own, continue mouth-to-mouth ventilation at the rate of 12 breaths per minute. THE ONLY WAY TO LEARN THIS TECHNIQUE IS TO TAKE A CPR COURSE — IT CANNOT BE PROPERLY SELF-TAUGHT.

CARDIAC COMPRESSION — Touch the victim and loudly ask if they are ok. If the victim is unresponsive, check their carotid pulse. This is easily found by placing your hand on the voice box (larynx). Slide the tips of your fingers into the groove beside the voice box and feel for the pulse — this is where the carotid artery can easily be felt. If the pulse cannot be felt, the rescuer must provide artificial circulation in addition to rescue breathing.

This is best done by external chest compression (see figure 27A&B). Kneel at the victim's side near his chest, locating the notch at the lowest portion of his breast bone or sternum. Place the heel of one hand on the sternum 1 1/2 to 2 inches above this notch. Place the other hand on top of the one that is in position on the sternum. Be sure to keep your fingers off of the ribs. The easiest way to prevent this is to interlock your fingers, thus keeping them confined to the sternum.

With your shoulders directly over the victim's sternum, compress downward keeping your arms straight. Depress the sternum 1 1/2 to 2 inches for an average adult victim. Relax the pressure completely, keeping your hands in contact with the sternum at all times, but allowing the sternum to return to its normal position between compressions. Both compression and relaxation should be of equal duration.

Perform 15 external chest compressions at a rate of 80 to 100 per minute. Open the airway and deliver 2 rescue breaths. Locate the proper hand position and begin 15 more compressions at a rate of 80 to 100 per minute. Perform 4 complete cycles of 15 compressions and 2 ventilations.

After 4 cycles of compressions and ventilations (15:2 ration), reevaluate the patient. Check for the return of the carotid pulse (5 seconds). If it is absent, resume CPR with 2 ventilations followed by compressions. If it is present, continue to the next step.

Check breathing (3 to 5 seconds). If present, monitor breathing and pulse closely. If absent, perform rescue breathing at 12 times per minute and monitor pulse closely.

If CPR is continued, stop and check for return of pulse and spontaneous breathing every few minutes. Do not interrupt CPR for more than 7 seconds except in special circumstances.

Once CPR is started it should be maintained until professional assistance can take over the responsibility, or until a physician declares the patient dead. If CPR has been continued for 30 minutes without regaining cardiac function, and the eyes are fixed and non-reactive to light, the patient can be presumed dead. The exceptions would be hypothermia and lightning injuries. In these circumstances CPR should be continued until the rescuers are exhausted if professional help does not intervene.

Immediately starting CPR and continuing it for as long as possible is the only possible chance for survival that a person has from potential drowning, cold water submersion, or lightning strike injury. Some authorities in wilderness rescue have felt that the survival rate is so low without defibrillation within 4 minutes by paramedics, that CPR should not be started in the bush when cardiac standstill is due to a heart attack. It certainly should not be started or maintained under conditions when its performance might endanger the lives of members of the rescue party.

Learning CPR is an important skill that every person should master. THE ONLY WAY TO LEARN THIS TECHNIQUE IS TO TAKE A CPR COURSE — IT CANNOT BE PROPERLY SELF-TAUGHT.

FOREIGN-BODY AIRWAY OBSTRUCTION MAN-EUVERS — The subdiaphragmatic abdominal thrust, also called "Abdominal thrust" or "Heimlich Maneuver," is recommended for relieving foreign-body airway obstruction, or choking. If the victim is standing or sitting, the rescuer stands behind and wraps his arms around the patient, proceeding as follows: Make a fist with one hand. Place the thumb side of the fist against the victim's abdomen, in the midline slightly above the navel and well below the breast bone (xiphoid process of the sternum). Grasp the fist with the other hand. Press the fist into the victim's abdomen with a quick upward thrust. Each new thrust should be a separate and distinct movement. It may be necessary to repeat the thrust 6 to 10 times to clear the airway.

If the victim is unconscious or on the ground, the victim should be placed on his back face up. The rescuer kneels astride the victim's thighs. The rescuer places the heel of one hand against the victim's abdomen, in the midline slightly above the navel and well below the breast bone, and the second hand directly on top of the fist. The rescuer then presses into the abdomen with a quick upward thrust.

APPENDIX B

The Outdoor First Aid Kit

State-of-the-art dressings, wound closure tapes, and non-prescription medications allow the construction of a very useful first aid kit for general outdoor use.

This book has described various first aid procedures that frequently use the items listed in the following kit. Very often treatments can be improvised with other items on hand, but prior planning and the inclusion of these items in your kit will provide you with the best that modern medical science can offer.

This kit, and all of the individual components, are available from Indiana Camp Supply, as indicated below.

Quantity	Item
2 pkgs	Coverstrip Closures ¼" x 3" 3/pkg
1	Spenco 2nd Skin Dressing Kit
1	Bulb irrigating syringe
5 pkg	Nu-Gauze, high absorbent, sterile, 2 ply, 3" x 3" pkg/2

1	Surgipad, Sterile, 8" x 10"
2	Elastomull, Sterile Roller Gauze, 4" x 162"
2	Elastomull, Sterile Roller Gauze, 2½" x 162"
10	Coverlet Bandage Strips 1" x 3"
1	Tape, Hypoallergenic ½" x 10 YD
1	Hydrocortisone Cream .5%, 1 oz tube (allergic skin)
1	Triple Antibiotic Ointment, 1 oz tube (prevents infection)
1	Hibiclens Surgical Scrub, 4 oz (prevents infection)
1	Dibucaine Ointment 1%, 1 oz tube (local pain relief)
1	Tetrahydrozoline Ophthalmic Drops, (eye irritation)
1	Starr Otic Drops, ½ oz bottle (ear pain, wax)
1	Micronazole Cream, 2%, ½ oz tube (fungal infection)
24	Actifed Tablets (decongestant)
24	Mobigesic Tablets (pain, fever, inflammation)
24	Meclizine 25 mg tab (nausea, motion sickness prevention)
2	Ammonia Inhalants (stimulant)
24	Benadryl 25 mg cap (antihistamine)
10	Bisacodyl 5 mg (constipation)
25	Diasorb (diarrhea)
25	Dimacid (antacid)
2 pkg	Q-tips, sterile, 2 per package
1	Extractor Kit (snake bite, sting, wound care)
6	1 oz Vials for repackaging the above
1	Over-pak Container for above

Consideration should be given to a dental kit. Several are commercially available through backpacking and outdoor outfitters. As a minimum, a small bottle of oil of cloves can serve as a topical

toothache treatment or a tube of toothache gel can be obtained. A
fever thermometer should be included on trips. People wearing
contact lenses should carry suction cup or rubber pincher device to
aid in their removal. An adequate means of water purification must
also be arranged.

Additional modules to this kit are described in detail in reference 5, some of which include prescription level medications. The
above kit, and the advanced treatment modules, can be purchased
pre-packed, and /or the individual items may be purchased sepa-
rately from Indiana Camp Supply, Inc., PO Box 211, Hobart,
Indiana 46342 — telephone (219) 947-2525.

APPENDIX C

Water Purification

Water can be purified adequately for drinking by mechanical, physical, and chemical means. The most clear water possible should be chosen, or attempts made to clarify the water, prior to starting any disinfectant process. Water with high particulate count or clay, or organic debris, allows higher bacterial counts and tends to be more heavily contaminated. When using chemical methods, cold water must be allowed to stand in contact longer to allow adequate reaction times. In preparing potable, or drinkable, water we are attempting to lower disease causing micro-organism counts to the point that the body can defend itself against the remaining numbers. We are not trying to produce sterile water, that would generally be impractical.

Chemical Purification Methods

Substance	Amount Used	Contact Time
Laundry Bleach 4-6%	2 drops/quart	Let stand 30 minutes

   (water should have a slight chlorine odor; if not, repeat dose and let stand an additional 15 minutes)

Halazone Tablets	5 tablets/quart	Let stand 30 minutes

   (defective Halazone tablets have an objectionable odor)

Tincture of Iodine 2% 10 drops/qt cloudy water	5 drops/qt clear water	30 minutes
Potable Aqua (Globuline - Tetraglycine hydroperiodide)	1 tablet/qt clear water 1 tab/qt cloudy water if very cold	10 minutes 20 minutes 30 minutes

Crystals of iodine can also be used to prepare a saturated iodine-water solution for use in disinfecting drinking water. Four to eight grams of USP grade iodine crystals can be placed in a 1 ounce glass bottle. Water added to this bottle will dissolve an amount of iodine based upon its temperature. It is this saturated iodine-water solution which is then added to the quart of water. The amount added to produce a final concentration of 4 ppm will vary according to temperature as indicated in the chart:

TEMPERATURE	VOLUME	CAPFULS*
37°F (3°C)	20.0 cc	8
68°F (20°C)	13.0 cc	5+
77°F (25°C)	12.5 cc	5
104°F (40°C)	10.0 cc	4

*Assuming 2½cc capacity for a standard 1 ounce glass bottle cap.

This water should be stored for 15 minutes before drinking. If the water is turbid, or otherwise contaminated, the amounts of saturated iodine solution indicated above should be doubled and the resultant water stored 20 minutes before using. This product is now commercially available as Polar Pure through many outdoor stores and catalog houses.

Filter systems exist, but water should be pre-treated before using to prevent filter contamination. An exception is the ceramic filter, the Katadyn Pocket Filter system, which while it will not become contaminated will become plugged and require occasional scraping with a special brush.

Bringing water to a boil will effectively kill germs and make water safe to drink. One reads variously to boil water 5, 10, even 20 minutes. But simply bringing the water temperature to 150°F

(65.5°C) is adequate to kill all water borne germs. At high altitude the boiling point of water is reduced. For example, at 25,000 feet the boiling point of water would be about 185°F (85°C), still quite adequate to prepare safe drinking water.

APPENDIX D

Bibliography

1. AUERBACH, PAUL, *Medicine for the Outdoors*, Little, Brown and Co., Boston, 1986.

2. DARVILL, FRED, *Mountaineering Medicine, 11th Edition*, Wilderness Press, Berkely, 1985.

3. EISENBERG, MICKEY and MICHAEL COPASS, *Manual of Emergency Medical Therapeutics*, W. B. Saunders Company, Philadelphia, 1978.

4. FORGEY, WILLIAM, *Hypothermia: Death by Exposure*, ICS Books, Merrillville, IN 1985.

5. FORGEY, WILLIAM, *Wilderness Medicine, 3rd Edition*, ICS Books, Merrillville, IN, 1987.

6. GOODMAN, PHILIP, et al, "Medical Recommendations for Wilderness Travel Part 3 — Medical Supplies and Drug Regimens," Postgraduate Medicine, *Vol 78, No 2, page 107, August 1985.*

7. GOODMAN, PHILIP, draft chapter on "Wilderness Emergency Medical Equipment" in AUERBACH, PAUL and EDWARD GEEHR, *Management of Wilderness and Environmental Emergencies*, Macmillan, New York, due in 1988.

8. LENTZ, MARTHA, et al, *Mountaineering First Aid, 3rd Edition*, Mountaineers, Seattle, 1985.

9. NELSON, RICHARD, et al., *Environmental Emergencies*, W. B. Saunders Company, Philadelphia, 1985.

10. WILKERSON, JAMES (Ed), *Medicine for Mountaineering, 3rd Edition*, Mountaineers, Seattle, 1985.

11. WILKERSON, JAMES (Ed), *Hypothermia, Frostbite and Other Cold Injuries*, Mountaineers, Seattle, 1986.

INDEX

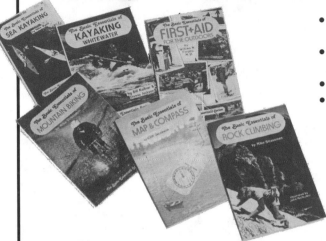
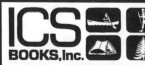